BRAIN HEALTH RECIPES

"FINDING THE BEST DIET FOR A HEALTHY BRAIN IN ALZHEIMER'S CARE"

Mark J. Schmitt

All right reserved. Do not republish any part of this publication in any form or by any means, including scanning, photocopying, or otherwise, without prior written permission from the copyright holder.

Copyright© Mark J. Schmitt

TABLE OF CONTENT

CHAPTER ONE 4
INTRODUCTION 4
CHAPTER TWO 8
THE ALZHEIMER'S DIET BASICS 8
CHAPTER THREE 13
BREAKFAST IS GOOD FOR YOU 13
    Breakfast Meal 13
CHAPTER FOUR 19
LUNCHES THAT ARE GOOD FOR YOU 19
    Lunch Meal 19
CHAPTER FIVE 25
WHOLESOME DINNERS 25
    Dinner Meal 25
        Vegetarian chili 29
CHAPTER SIX 32
HEALTHY SNACKS 32
    Greek yogurt 35
CHAPTER SEVEN 38
HYDRATION STATION 38
    Relaxing Herbal Teas 40
        Fresh herbs like mint and basil 42
CHAPTER EIGHT 44
DESSERTS WITH A TWIST 44
CHAPTER NINE 50
RECIPES FOR SPECIAL OCCASIONS 50
CHAPTER TEN 56
KITCHEN TIPS AND TECHNIQUES 56
CHAPTER ELEVEN 62
CAREGIVER'S CORNER 62
CHAPTER TWELVE 67
CONCLUSION 67

CHAPTER ONE

INTRODUCTION

This Cookbook Can Help Alzheimer's Patients Eat Healthy.
Care of what people with Alzheimer's eat requires good planning and understanding. This cookbook includes recipes and offers useful advice for eating healthy to help people with Alzheimer's. This cookbook is useful.

- Personalized recipes for brain health.
Choosing ingredients carefully: Every recipe uses ingredients that are good for your brain, helping it work better and keeping you healthy.

- Simple and user-friendly.
Easy Instructions: Recipes have simple, step-by-step directions that are easy for caregivers and people with Alzheimer's to understand.
Easy: Cooking meals without stress by keeping it simple.

Different types of food and how to eat well.
You can pick from different recipes: We offer a variety of dishes from different meals and cuisines to help you have a healthy and tasty diet.
Full of nutrients: Picking foods that provide your body with what it needs to be healthy.

- Dealing with food problems.
Adaptability: Providing recipes that can be modified to assist with common eating issues for people with Alzheimer's, such as altering the texture of the food.
Better Nutrition: Ensure every recipe includes plenty of healthy nutrients for different diets.

Using the Senses
Nice Presentation: Knowing how important it is to make food look appealing and catch people's eye.
Making food more appealing: Using tasty flavors and nice smells to make people want to eat more.

- Caregiver Support
Tips for caregivers: This includes ideas on how to plan and make meals, and how to help others eat healthy.
Considering your preferences: Offering options to change meals to fit what you like.

-Promoting Social Interaction
Eating Together: We think that sharing meals with others and enjoying their company is helpful for our mental well-being.
Making Good Memories: Picking recipes that bring back happy memories to improve the eating experience.

This cookbook has recipes that help you eat healthy meals for people with Alzheimer's. It aims to help people enjoy eating and feel good by focusing on thinking skills, keeping things easy, offering different kinds of food, and supporting caregivers.

People with Alzheimer's need to eat healthy food.
Alzheimer's disease is a complicated brain condition that affects memory, thinking, and eating. Understanding how important it is to eat the right foods when you have Alzheimer's is really important for making people's lives better.

- Support for thinking and mental processes.
Eating the right foods can help your brain work better. Nutrients like omega-3 fatty acids and antioxidants play an important role in keeping your brain healthy.
Slowing Down Memory Loss: Studying how eating healthy can help to slow down memory loss in people with Alzheimer's disease.

-Physical health means taking care of your body.
It's about eating well, exercising, and staying healthy. When you take care of your physical health, you feel good in your body and mind.
Managing your weight:
Dealing with the difficulties of losing or gaining weight that come with Alzheimer's disease and how it affects your overall health. Ensuring you drink enough water is crucial for maintaining your body's health.

-Staying independent
Eating well helps you do things on your own.
Improving Life: How eating the right foods can make life better for people with Alzheimer's.

-Problems and ways to fix them
Helping people with Alzheimer's disease with their eating problems by understanding what difficulties they might have and finding ways to help them eat better.

-Personalized Nutrition Plans:
Making food plans that fit individual likes and needs.

-Help and advice for caregivers.
Teaching caregivers about how to help people with Alzheimer's and making sure they have the right information and tools to meet their nutritional needs.
Working with doctors and nurses to make good diet plans is very important.

- Making life better.
The way you eat can make you feel happy and have a good effect on your emotions and thoughts.

Helping people with Alzheimer's disease feel good and respected by giving them good food and making sure they are comfortable.
it's important to understand and meet the nutritional needs of people with Alzheimer's as part of their overall care. By paying attention to what we eat, we can help people with Alzheimer's disease to think better, stay healthy, and have a good life.

CHAPTER TWO

THE ALZHEIMER'S DIET BASICS

What is the diet for Alzheimer's?
Understanding the idea.
Alzheimer's disease is a brain problem that gets worse as time goes on and people want to know if certain foods can help improve thinking and memory. The Alzheimer's Diet is a way of eating that helps people with Alzheimer's disease keep their brains healthy and slow down memory loss. It also makes them feel better.

Important Nutrients for Brain Health
Many vitamins and minerals help keep the brain healthy and may lower the chance of losing mental abilities. Eating a mix of different foods is the best way to make sure you get all the nutrients you need. Here are some important nutrients that help keep your brain healthy:

Omega-3 fatty acids:
are good for your brain and you can find them in fish like salmon, mackerel, and trout, as well as in flax seeds, chai seeds, and walnuts.

They might help us think and protect against memory loss as we get older.

Antioxidants :This substance can help keep the brain safe from harm that can lead to memory and thinking issues. Foods such as berries, oranges, leafy vegetables, nuts, and seeds contain antioxidants.

Vitamins:
Nutrients that our bodies need to be healthy.
Vitamin E is found in nuts, seeds, spinach, and other green leafy vegetables. It helps keep your brain strong.
Meat, fish, and dairy products are sources of Vitamin B12. It helps create red blood cells and keeps the nervous system in good shape.
Fol ate (Vitamin B9) is found in leafy vegetables, beans, and some grains that have added nutrients. It helps with thinking and memory.

Minerals:
Minerals are naturally occurring substances that exist in the earth.
Iron is the key to transporting oxygen throughout the body. You can find iron in meat, beans, lentils, and fortified cereals.
Zinc can be found in meat, dairy, nuts, and legumes, and it helps with the brain and nerves.
Magnesium is in foods like spinach, nuts, and whole grains. It helps keep your brain healthy.
Phosphor lipids: Choline helps make a chemical called acetylcholine, which is important for memory and learning in the brain. Some foods that have choline are eggs, meat, and some kinds of beans.

Curcumin is a compound in turmeric that helps reduce inflammation and works as an antioxidant. Some research shows it might be good for thinking and memory.

Flavonoid are natural substances found in foods like berries, citrus fruits, tea, and dark chocolate. They have antioxidants and help reduce inflammation in the body, which can be good for the brain.

Keep in mind that some nutrients may help prevent or treat memory loss, but more research is needed to know for sure.

Foods to Eat and Not Eat

When thinking about what to eat for brain health, it is important to eat a variety of healthy foods. Here are some general rules about food, but everyone's needs are different. It's best to talk to a doctor or a nutrition expert for personalized advice.

Foods that are good for the brain:
Fatty Fish: Oily Fish:
Full of omega-3 fatty acids, which are important for keeping the brain healthy. Some examples are salmon, mackerel, trout, and sardines.

Berries:
Small, round fruits that are usually sweet and can be eaten fresh or used in cooking and baking. Included in the examples are strawberries, blueberries, raspberries, and blackberries.
Full of powerful nutrients that can help your brain work better. Blueberries, strawberries, and blackberries are healthy options.

Green vegetables:
Green plants and leafy vegetables.
Packed with vitamins, minerals, and healthy stuff. Some green leafy vegetables are spinach, kale, and Swiss chard.

Nuts and seeds:
Healthy foods with omega-3 fats, antioxidants, and vitamin E. Almonds, walnuts, chia seeds, and flax seeds are good for you.

Whole Grains:
Whole grains are foods that are made from the entire grain, including the bran, germ, and endosperm. They provide important nutrients and fiber that are good for your health. Whole grains are foods such as brown rice, quinoa, and wheat bread.

Give the brain a constant flow of energy. Pick foods like brown rice, quinoa, oats, and whole wheat.

Avocado
Avocado: a fruit with green skin and a large seed inside.
Has good fats that help the brain stay healthy.

Broccoli
Broccoli is a green vegetable that is good for you.
Rich in antioxidants and vitamin K, which is good for the brain.

Eggs:
Eggs: Eggs are a type of food that comes from birds, like chickens. They are a great source of protein and can be prepared in many ways.
Choline is important for making a chemical called acetylcholine, which helps with memory and mood.

Turmeric
Turmeric is a plant with a bright yellow root that is often used as a spice in cooking and for its health benefits.
Contains curcumin, which helps to reduce inflammation and acts as an antioxidant. It is a popular seasoning in curry recipes.

Dark chocolate
Dark chocolate is a type of chocolate that has a high percentage of cocoa and a rich, intense flavor.
Has substances called flavonoid and caffeine that make your memory and thinking better. Pick dark chocolate that has 70% cocoa or more.

Green tea
Full of antioxidants, like catechins, that could protect the brain.

Bright and colorful veggies:
Bell peppers, tomatoes, and carrots have lots of good stuff like vitamins and antioxidants.

Foods that you should consider reducing consumption of or staying away from.

Processed Foods:
Food that has been changed from its original form through cooking, packaging, or adding ingredients.
This has a lot of sugar, bad fats, and preservatives. These things can cause swelling and may harm the way the brain works.

Trans fats
Trans fats are a type of unhealthy fat that can raise your bad (LDL) cholesterol levels and increase your risk of heart disease. They are often found in processed foods like fried items, baked goods, and snacks. It's important to limit trans fats in your diet to stay healthy.
Seen in lots of pre-made and cooked foods. Trans fats can negatively impact brain function and are detrimental to brain health.

Sodas and other sweet drinks:
Eating a lot of sugar has been connected to a decrease in thinking abilities. Pick water, herbal teas, or drinks without extra sugars.

Highly processed carbohydrates:
Eat less white bread, pastries, and sugary cereals. Pick whole grains that have not been processed.

Too much drinking of alcohol:
Drinking a little alcohol might be good for you, but drinking too much can hurt your thinking skills.

Foods with a lot of salt:
Eating too much salt can make your blood pressure go up, and that can affect how well your brain works.

CHAPTER THREE

BREAKFAST IS GOOD FOR YOU

Eating a healthy breakfast is important for giving you the energy and nutrients you need to start your day and keep your body and brain working well. Here are some suggestions for breakfast that can help give you more energy and help you concentrate better.

Breakfast Meal
Blueberry Oatmeal Muffins
Muffins made with blueberries and oats.
Blueberry oat muffins are a yummy and healthy choice for breakfast or a snack.

Basic recipe

Ingredients:
1 cup of oats that are traditional and rolled.
1 cup of either white flour or whole wheat flour

1/2 cup of brown sugar that has been pressed down firmly
1 small spoon of baking powder
Half a teaspoon of baking soda
One half of a small spoon of salt.
1 measuring cup of regular Greek yogurt
1/4th cup of butter that does not have salt in it, which is melted and then left to cool.
One big egg
1 small spoonful of vanilla flavor
Use 1 cup of fresh or frozen blueberries.
Here are the steps to follow:
First, heat the oven.

Heat your oven to 375°F (190°C) before you start cooking. Put paper liners in the muffin tin or grease the cups.

Make oatmeal:
Mix the oats with the Greek yogurt in a bowl. Allow the oats to sit for 10 minutes to get soft.
Mix all the dry ingredients.

In a big bowl, mix the flour, brown sugar, baking powder, baking soda, and salt.

Mix the wet ingredients.
Put the melted butter, egg, and vanilla extract in the bowl with the oats and yogurt. Stir until everything is mixed well.

Mix wet and dry ingredients.
Mix the wet ingredients with the dry ones and gently stir until combined. Be cautious not to mix too much; it's fine if there are a few lumps.
Introduce blueberries:

Carefully mix the blueberries into the batter so they are spread out evenly. Put the batter into the muffin cups.

Put the batter into the muffin cups until they are about 2/3 full.

Cook in the oven.

Put the muffins in the oven that has been heated beforehand and leave them in for 18-22 minutes. Check if they are ready by poking a toothpick into the middle of a muffin - if it comes out clean or with a few wet crumbs on it, then the muffins are ready.
Awesome

Let the muffins cool in the tin for 5 minutes, then put them on a rack to cool completely.
Have fun:

After they cool down, you can enjoy these blueberry oatmeal muffins as a yummy and healthy snack.
You can change the recipe by putting a little bit of oats or a small amount of cinnamon on top before you bake it. You can use some whole wheat flour instead of regular flour to make it healthier. Change how sweet it is by adding more or less brown sugar.

Wraps with spinach and feta cheese
Spinach and feta breakfast wraps are a delicious and healthy way to begin your day. Here's an easy way to make tasty spinach and feta breakfast wraps:

Ingredients:
Whole-grain or wraps flavored with spinach.
4 big eggs
1 cup of fresh spinach leaves that have been cleaned and cut into smaller pieces.
Half a cup of crumbled feta cheese
1 spoonful of olive oil
Put salt and pepper as much as you desire to make it taste good.
You can add diced tomatoes, avocado slices, salsa, or hot sauce if you want.

Rules: I will provide you with directions.
Get all the things you need to cook.

Clean and cut the fresh spinach.
Cut the feta cheese into little bits.

Cook spinach in a pan with oil or butter.
Warm the olive oil in a pan on a medium heat. Put the cut spinach in the pan and cook for 1-2 minutes until it gets soft. Add a little bit of salt and pepper until it tastes good.

Make scrambled eggs:
In a bowl, mix the eggs. Put the mixed eggs into the pan with the cooked spinach.

Make eggs in a pan.
Scramble the eggs in a pan, stirring gently, until they are fully cooked. This will take 2-3 minutes.

Include some feta cheese:
Put the broken feta cheese on top of the eggs. Let it start to melt while you keep stirring.

Warm Wraps:
In a different pan or directly on the stove, heat the wraps for 10-15 seconds on each side.

Make Wraps:
Put the scrambled eggs, spinach, and feta mixture in the middle of each warm wrap.

Add extra ingredients on top of the main food item.
You can add toppings like tomatoes, avocado, salsa, or hot sauce if you want.

Wrap and Serve:
Wrap and Serve means to wrap something up, like a sandwich or a present, and then give it to someone.
Fold the edges of the wrap over the filling and then roll it up from the bottom to make a wrap. If needed, use a toothpick to keep it in place.

Have fun:

Your spinach and feta breakfast wraps are ready to eat. Serve the food to them while it is hot.
You can change the recipe by adding things like cooked mushrooms, onions, or peppers. Also, you can pick flavored wraps or tortillas to add different tastes. These wraps can be used in many ways and are a good choice for a fast and healthy breakfast.

Healthy breakfast option with lots of nutrients: Smoothie Bowls
Smoothie bowls are a tasty and healthy breakfast option that gives you a lot of vitamins and energy. Here's a simple recipe for a healthy smoothie bowl that you can make just the way you like it.

Ingredients:
For the smoothie base:
1 banana that is frozen and cut into pieces.
1 measured cup of frozen berries mixed (like strawberries, blueberries, and raspberries)
1/2 cup of regular Greek yogurt.
1/2 cup of spinach or kale leaves, either fresh or frozen.
1/2 cup of almond milk or your favorite type of milk.
1 spoon of chia seeds or flaxseeds (if you want more fiber)
1 teaspoon of honey or maple syrup (if you want to add some sweetness)

Toppings:
Cut up fruits like berries, bananas, and kiwi.
Granola is a type of breakfast cereal made from rolled oats, nuts, honey, and sometimes dried fruits.
Nuts and seeds such as almonds, walnuts, chia seeds, and pumpkin seeds.
Grated coconut
Grated coconut with a hint of honey or nut butter.

Steps:
Get the ingredients ready for putting on top of the food.
Cut up the fresh fruits for the top of the dish.
Weigh out granola, nuts, seeds, and other toppings.

Mix Smoothie Starter:
Put frozen bananas, frozen berries, Greek yogurt, spinach or kale, almond milk, and chia or flaxseeds in a blender and mix them.
Mix until it becomes smooth and creamy. If the mixture is too hard, you can add a little more almond milk.

Pour the contents into a bowl.
Put the smoothie in a bowl.
Add extra ingredients on top of your food.
Put the cut fruits, granola, nuts, seeds, and shredded coconut on the smoothie.

Drizzle some honey or spread some nut butter.
You can add some honey or nut butter on top for more flavor if you want.
Have fun:

Get a spoon and enjoy your healthy smoothie bowl.
Advice for customizing something:
Add a little protein powder to the smoothie if you want to have more protein in it.

Different types of liquid can be used such as coconut water, plain water, or milk depending on what you like.

Try using different leafy greens like kale, spinach, or chard for more nutrients.

Different types of frozen fruits: You can use any combination of frozen fruits that you like or have on hand.

You can use lots of different ingredients and toppings to make delicious smoothie bowls. Go ahead and be creative and try new things. They not only look good but also provide lots of important vitamins and minerals to start your day off right.

CHAPTER FOUR

LUNCHES THAT ARE GOOD FOR YOU

Making healthy lunches means having the right mix of proteins, carbs, and fats, as well as getting different vitamins and minerals. Here are some lunch ideas with good nutrients.

Lunch Meal
Salmon and Avocado Salad
A salad with salmon and avocado is a tasty and healthy choice for lunch. Here is an easy way to make tasty Salmon.

Avocado Salad:
a salad made with avocados.
Ingredients: List of things used to make something.
For the fish that is called salmon:
2 pieces of salmon (fresh or cooked).
1 spoon of olive oil
Add salt and pepper to your liking.
Sliced lemons for squeezing.

For the salad:

Various types of lettuce (such as spinach, arugula, or a mix of different types)
1 ripe avocado, cut into slices
Cut the cherry tomatoes in half.
Cut the cucumber into slices.
Cut the red onion into thin slices.

To make the dressing:
2 tablespoons of really good olive oil
1 tablespoon of balsamic vinegar
1 small spoon of Dijon mustard
The amount of salt and pepper you use is up to your personal preference.

Follow the steps:
Get the salmon ready:
If the salmon isn't cooked, heat the oven to 400°F (200°C).
Put the salmon pieces on a baking tray, pour some olive oil over them, and sprinkle with salt and pepper.
Cook the salmon in the oven for 12-15 minutes until it is cooked and easy to break apart with a fork. You can also cook the salmon on a grill or in a pan.

Make the salad:
In a big bowl, mix the salad greens, avocado, tomatoes, cucumber, and onion.

Prepare the dressing:
Mix the olive oil, balsamic vinegar, Dijon mustard, salt, and pepper in a small bowl until they are well mixed.

Make the salad.
Cut the cooked salmon into small pieces and put it in the salad.
Pour the dressing on the salad and mix it carefully so that all the ingredients are covered evenly.

Serve:
Split the salad onto separate plates or bowls.
Squeeze lemon on the salmon for more freshness.
Have fun

Your salad with salmon and avocado is all done and you can have it for a tasty and satisfying lunch.

Optional extras: optional things you can add on if you want to.
Add cooked quinoa or farro to make the salad more filling.

Nuts or Seeds: Add some toasted pine nuts, almonds, or pumpkin seeds for extra crunch.

Use some crumbled feta or goat cheese on top of the salad for more taste.

You can change the recipe to fit your tastes and dietary needs. This salad has good fats, protein, and lots of vitamins and minerals.

Stuffed Peppers with Quinoa and Vegetables
Quinoa and vegetables inside peppers make a healthy and filling meal. Here's an easy way to make stuffed peppers with **quinoa and vegetables:**

Ingredients:
4 big bell peppers (any color)
1 cup of quinoa, washed and cooked as per the instructions on the package.
1 spoonful of olive oil
1 onion, cut into small pieces.
2 pieces of garlic, finely chopped
1 zucchini, cut into small pieces
One carrot, shredded into small pieces.
Half a cup of cherry tomatoes.
1 cup of black beans, remove the liquid and wash them.
1 teaspoon of powdered cumin
1 small spoon of paprika
Put salt and pepper as you desire.
1 cup of cheese that is shredded. It can be cheddar, mozzarella, or any other type you prefer.
Fresh parsley or cilantro for decoration

Steps to follow:
Preheat the oven.
Set your oven to 375 degrees Fahrenheit and let it heat up.

Prepare for the bell peppers.

Get ready for the bell peppers:
Cut off the tops of the bell peppers and take out the seeds and insides. Gently spread a little bit of olive oil on the outside of the peppers.
Make Quinoa:

Prepare quinoa as directed on the package. Put to the side.

Cook vegetables in a pan with some oil over medium heat, stirring them frequently until they are tender.
In a big pan, warm up the olive oil on medium heat. Cook the chopped onion and garlic in a pan until they are soft.
Put chopped zucchini, grated carrot, cherry tomatoes, and black beans in the pan. Continue cooking for another 5-7 minutes until the vegetables are soft.

Flavor the mix:
Mix in powdered cumin, paprika, and a little bit of salt and pepper. Season it how you like it.

Mix with Quinoa:
Stir the cooked quinoa with the sautéed vegetables. Let it cool down a little. Fill the peppers with ingredients of your choice.

Put the quinoa and vegetable mixture inside each bell pepper. Gently push the filling into the peppers and sprinkle cheese on top.

Cook in an oven.
Put the stuffed peppers in a baking pan. Put the peppers in the hot oven and cook for 25-30 minutes until they are soft and the cheese on top is melted and golden.
Garnish means to decorate or add something extra to a dish, usually for added flavor or visual appeal.

Sprinkle with fresh parsley or cilantro.

Serve:
Please serve the hot quinoa and vegetable stuffed peppers. You can eat them alone or with a salad.
Extra things you can choose to include:
Add cooked ground turkey, chicken, or tofu to the quinoa and vegetables to

get more protein.

Spices: Add your favorite spices or herbs to make the flavor just right for you.

You can change the ingredients and seasonings in this recipe to make it taste how you like. Quinoa and vegetable stuffed peppers are a healthy meal with lots of protein, fiber, and important nutrients.

Chicken and Broccoli Stir-Fry

Chicken and broccoli stir-fry is a fast and tasty meal that is both filling and good for you. Here's an easy way to make a dish with chicken and broccoli.

Ingredients list:
1 pound of boneless, skinless chicken breasts that are sliced thinly (about 450 grams)
4 cups of chopped broccoli.
2 spoons of soy sauce (low-sodium if you like)
1 spoonful of oyster sauce
1 spoon of hoisin sauce
1 spoonful of rice vinegar
1 spoon of sesame oil
2 tablespoons of oil made from plants (for cooking)
3 pieces of garlic, chopped finely
1 small spoon of fresh ginger, finely chopped
2 spoons of water
Sesame seeds and chopped green onions for decoration (if you want).

Cooked rice or noodles for serving
"Steps to follow:"
Get the chicken ready:
Cut the chicken breasts into thin pieces and keep them aside.

Cook the broccoli in boiling water for a short time.
Bring a pot of water to a boil. Cook the broccoli in boiling water for 2-3 minutes until they are a bright green color. Pour out the liquid and put it to the side.

Prepare the stir-fry sauce:
In a small bowl, mix soy sauce, oyster sauce, hoisin sauce, rice vinegar, and

sesame oil and put it aside.

Cook Chicken:
Warm up the vegetable oil in a wok or big frying pan on medium-high heat. Put the sliced chicken in and cook it until it is fully cooked and has a light brown color. Take out the chicken from the pan and keep it to the side.

Cook Garlic and Ginger:
Include a small oil to the pan if desired. Mix in chopped garlic and grated ginger. Cook in a hot pan for about 30 seconds or until it starts to smell good.

Add some broccoli and chicken.
Put the broccoli and chicken back in the pan.

Add the sauce.
Put the sauce on the chicken and broccoli. Mix 2 spoonfuls of water with the sauce to spread it out evenly.

Stir-Fry:
An easy way to cook vegetables and meat quickly in a hot pan with oil.
Cook the ingredients in a pan for 2-3 minutes until they are covered in the sauce and heated.

Add a little decoration to make the dish look nice, then give it to the people to eat.

Sprinkle sesame seeds and chopped green onions on top if you like.

You can have it with rice or noodles.
Put the chicken and broccoli stir-fry on top of cooked rice or noodles.
Additional options that are not required.
Cashews or almonds: Put a few in for extra crunch.

Sprinkle red pepper flakes into the food while cooking to add some spiciness.

This chicken and broccoli stir-fry can be changed to how you like it. It's a good meal with meat, veggies, and tasty sauce.

CHAPTER FIVE

WHOLESOME DINNERS

Making healthy dinners means including a good mix of proteins, carbohydrates, and fats, as well as different vitamins and minerals. Here are some healthy dinner ideas:

Dinner Meal
Simple Baked Cod with Lemon and Herbs
Baked cod with lemon and herbs is an easy and tasty dish that is both light and delicious. Here is an easy recipe for cooking baked cod:

Ingredients:
4. pieces of cod fish, each weighing about 6 ounces.
2 tablespoons of olive oil
2 tablespoons of freshly squeezed lemon juice.
2 pieces of garlic, chopped into very small pieces
1 small spoon of dried oregano
1 small spoon of dried thyme
Feel free to season with salt and pepper to your liking.
Pieces of lemon to put on the side of the dish.

Freshly cut parsley for garnish.

Instructions:
Preheat the oven before you start cooking.
Preheat your oven to a temperature of 400 degrees Fahrenheit or 200 degrees Celsius.

Get the cod fillets ready:
Use paper towels to dry the cod fillets by patting them gently. Put them on a baking sheet that's covered with parchment paper or a little bit of oil.

Mix the Marinade:
Mix olive oil, lemon juice, garlic, oregano, thyme, salt, and pepper in a small bowl.

Prepare the fish by soaking it in a flavored liquid for some time before cooking.
Coat the cod fillets with the marinade so that both sides are covered evenly.

Bake the Cod:
Bake the cod in the hot oven for 12-15 minutes until it looks white and can be easily separated with a fork.

Garnish:
Take out the cooked cod from the oven and add lemon slices and chopped fresh parsley on top.

Serve:
Enjoy the cooked cod with your favorite sides like vegetables, quinoa, or salad.

Optional Additions:
Add cut cherry tomatoes to the baking sheet for a pop of fresh flavor.

Olives: Put some chopped olives on top of the cod before baking for a Mediterranean flavor.

Capers: To give more taste, put capers in the marinade or sprinkle them on top of the cod before baking.

Here are some suggestions:
Even Thickness: Pick cod fillets that are the same thickness so they cook evenly.

Checking if the fish is cooked: The cod is cooked when it easily breaks apart with a fork. Be careful not to cook it for too long, or it will be dry.

This cooked cod with lemon and herbs goes well with many different side dishes. It's a healthy and easy choice for a tasty dinner.

Baked dish with turkey and sweet potatoes
Turkey and sweet potato casserole is a delicious and satisfying dish that mixes healthy meat with the natural sweetness of sweet potatoes. Here's an easy recipe to make a delicious turkey and sweet potato dish. Simple words: Here's a recipe to make a yummy turkey and sweet potato dish.

 Ingredients:
1 pound of ground turkey meat
Two big sweet potatoes, take off the skin and cut into thin pieces.
1 onion, cut into small pieces
Two pieces of garlic, chopped into small pieces.
1 cup of frozen peas
1 cup of chicken or turkey broth
1 cup of cheese that has been grated (either cheddar or mozzarella)
1 small spoonful of dried thyme
1 spoon of dried sage.
Use salt and pepper as much as you like.
Cooking with olive oil
Finely cut fresh parsley to sprinkle over the dish (if you want).

Here are the directions:
Preheat the oven: Heat the oven before using it.
Bring your oven up to 375Â°F or 190Â°C.

Make sweet potatoes ready:
Cut the sweet potatoes into thin slices after removing the skin. You can use a mandoline slicer to make slices even.

Make ground turkey in a pan.
Heat a little bit of olive oil in a big frying pan on medium heat. Cook the chopped onions and minced garlic in a pan until they are soft.
Put ground turkey in the pan and cook it until it turns brown. Use a spoon to break it into smaller pieces while cooking.

Spices the turkey.
Sprinkle dried thyme, dried sage, salt, and pepper on the turkey. Mix it well.

Include peas and broth:
Put frozen peas into the pan and pour in the turkey or chicken broth. Let the mixture cook for a few minutes until the peas are hot.

Put the casserole together:
In a buttered baking dish, arrange half of the sliced sweet potatoes in a layer.
Put the turkey mixture on top of the sweet potatoes using a spoon.
Put the rest of the sweet potatoes on the top.

Put cheese on top.
Put cheese on top of the casserole.

Serve:
Put foil on the dish and cook it in the oven for 30-40 minutes until the sweet potatoes are soft.

You can broil the food if you want to.
If you want the cheese to be brown and bubbly, take the lid off the pan and put it under the broiler for 3-5 minutes.

Garnish and Serve:
Add some chopped fresh parsley on top if you like. Allow it to sit for a little while before you serve it.

Optional Additions:

Cranberry Sauce:
Cranberry sauce is a sauce made from cranberries. It is sweet and can be served with turkey or other meats.
Serve with a little cranberry sauce on the side for a nice holiday touch.

Walnuts
Walnuts are nuts that grow on trees. They have a hard shell and a soft, tasty inside. People like to eat them as a snack or use them in cooking. They additionally contribute to maintaining your overall well-being.
Sprinkle chopped walnuts on top before baking for extra crunch.

This turkey and sweet potato dish has a good mix of protein, healthy carbs, and lots of delicious taste. Personalize it with the herbs and spices you like best.
Vegetarian Chili for a Cozy Evening

Vegetarian chili is a tasty and filling meal that's great for a comfortable night at home. Filled with beans, veggies, and tasty spices, it's a cozy and healthy choice. Here's a simple recipe for tasty vegetarian chili:

Ingredients:
2 spoons of olive oil
1 big onion, cut into small pieces.
3 pieces of garlic, chopped into small pieces
1 chopped bell pepper (any color)
Cut one zucchini into small pieces.
1 carrot, cut into small pieces
1 jalape, with the seeds removed and finely chopped (if you want it to be spicy)
One 15-ounce can of black beans, with the liquid poured out and then washed.
1 can of kidney beans (15 oz), drained and rinsed.
1 can of pinto beans that are 15 ounces, pour out the liquid, and wash the beans.
1 large can of grounded tomatoes (28 ounces)

1 cup of soup made from vegetables
2 spoons of tomato paste
2 teaspoons of powdered cumin.
2 small spoonfuls of chili powder.
1 small spoon of smoked paprika
1 small spoon of dried oregano
Put salt and pepper as you desire.
1 measure of frozen corn pieces
Fresh cilantro that is chopped up, to put on top as decoration.
Sliced avocado, for decoration (if wanted)
Cheese pieces, for adding (if you like)
You can use sour cream or Greek yogurt if you like.

Instructions:
Cook the vegetables in a little bit of oil over high heat, stirring often, until they are tender and slightly browned.
Heat olive oil in a pot on medium heat. Put chopped onion, garlic, pepper, squash, carrot, and spicy jalape. Keep the vegetables on the heat until they become soft.

Add Beans:
Put black beans, kidney beans, and pinto beans in the pot. Mix

Put the tomatoes and broth into the pot.
Put ground tomatoes, vegetable broth, and tomato paste in the pot. Mix thoroughly

Add seasoning to the chili to make it taste better.
Put cumin, chili powder, paprika, oregano, salt, and pepper. Mix

Simmer:
Heat the chili until it starts to bubble. Turn down the heat, put a lid on the pot, and let it cook gently for 20-30 minutes so the flavors can mix.

Put in some corn.
Add the frozen corn and let it cook for another 10-15 minutes.

Change the flavor to taste better.
Try the chili and add more salt or pepper if you think it needs it. Add more salt, pepper, or other spices to make it taste how you like it.

Serve:
Spoon the veggie chili into bowls. Sprinkle with chopped cilantro and add avocado slices, cheese, and a spoonful of sour cream or Greek yogurt if you like.

"Have fun"
Enjoy the vegetarian chili with some yummy bread for a delicious and comforting meal.
You can change the chili by adding more veggies, using different beans, or making it spicier to your liking. It's a dish that can be used in many ways and makes you feel good when it's cold outside.

CHAPTER SIX

HEALTHY SNACKS

Eating healthy snacks means picking foods with lots of nutrients, giving you energy, making you feel full, and helping you stay healthy. Here are some suggestions for snacks that are good for your health and are also smart choices.

Nut mix for hiking and snacking.
Making your nut mix lets you choose what nuts and flavors you like best, and what's healthiest for you. Here's an easy recipe for a healthy trail mix with nuts:

Ingredients:
1 cup of almonds
1 cup of walnuts
1 cup of cashew nuts.
1/2 a cup of pumpkin seeds
1/2 cup of sunflower seeds.
1/2 a cup of dried cranberries
Add in half a cup of dark chocolate chips or chunks.
1/2 teaspoon of sea salt (you can skip this if you prefer a sweeter taste)

Directions:
Preheat the oven (if you want).
Preheat the oven to 350°F (175°C) if you want to cook the nuts for more taste. it's optional.

You can optionally cook nuts by roasting them.
Place almonds, walnuts, and cashews on a baking pan. Cook in the hot oven for 8-10 minutes, stirring in the middle. Please remove it from the oven after baking and allow it to cool.

Mix the ingredients.
Mix the nuts, seeds, cranberries, and chocolate in a big bowl.

You may choose to add sea salt.
Put some sea salt on top if you want a mix of sweet and salty flavors. Mix thoroughly by tossing.

Keep in a tightly sealed container:
Put the nut trail mix into a container that closes tightly, or divide it into small bags for snacks.
"Have fun"

You can eat the nut trail mix by itself, put it on yogurt, or mix it with cereal.

Customization Tips:
Suggestions to make something unique to your liking.
Different: You can use different nuts and seeds like pistachios, pecans, or chia seeds if you want.

Try using different dried fruits like raisins, apricots, or blueberries to make your food sweeter.

Spices: Sprinkle a little bit of cinnamon, nutmeg, or your favorite spice mix to make the flavor even better.

Add some foods with a lot of protein, like roasted chickpeas or edamame, for an extra protein boost.

Making your nut mix lets you choose what you like, so you get the flavors and health benefits you want. It's a handy and easy-to-carry snack for a fast burst of energy.

Berries with creamy Greek yogurt
A tasty and healthy breakfast or snack is Greek yogurt with berries. Here's an easy way to make a delicious Greek yogurt parfait:

Ingredients:
1 cup of Greek yogurt, either plain or vanilla flavor.
1 cup of different types of berries (strawberries, blueberries, raspberries)
1/2 cup of crunchy oat and nut mixture.
1 spoon of honey or maple syrup (if you want it to be sweet)
You can add fresh mint leaves on top for decoration (if you want).

Instructions:
Get the berries ready:
Clean and get the berries ready. If you're using strawberries, remove the stem and cut them into slices.

Put Greek yogurt in a layer.
Put Greek yogurt in the bottom of a glass or bowl.

Include berries:
Put a bunch of berries on top of the yogurt.

Sprinkle the granola on top.
Put granola on top of the berries. You can use your choice of granola flavor to add variety and texture.

Repeat Layers:
Repeat the layers by putting more Greek yogurt, then berries, and then granola until the container is full.

Drizzle with honey, if you like.
If you want it sweeter, you can put honey or maple syrup on it.

Garnish with Mint (Optional):
Add some fresh mint leaves on top for a refreshing taste and a nice look.

Serve right away:
Put the Greek yogurt parfait on a plate and eat it right away. It's a yummy mix of smooth yogurt, fresh berries, and crispy granola.
Personalize your things by following these tips:
Nuts and Seeds: Sprinkle some nuts (like almonds or walnuts) or seeds (such as chia or pumpkin seeds) for extra crunch and health benefits.

Sprinkle a little bit of cinnamon or nutmeg on top of the parfait for more taste.

Dried fruits like raisins or dried cranberries give a chewy texture.

Sprinkle unsweetened coconut flakes on top for a tropical flavor.

Greek yogurt
This Greek yogurt parfait can be changed to fit what you like. It has protein, fiber, and antioxidants, so it's a healthy and filling choice for a fast and nutritious meal or snack.
Energy-Boosting Protein Bites

Energy-boosting protein bites are a handy and yummy way to get energized during the day. Here's an easy recipe for making protein bites that are full of good stuff and taste great:

Ingredients:
1 cup of the type of oats called old-fashioned oats.
1/2 cup of almond or peanut butter
1/3 cup of either honey or maple syrup.
Half a cup of protein powder, either vanilla or chocolate flavored.
1/2 cup of flaxseed that has been turned into a powder.
Half of a cup of dark chocolate chips.
1 small spoon of vanilla flavoring extracted from vanilla beans.
A little bit of salt

Directions:
Mix the dry stuff.
In a big bowl, stir together the oats, protein powder, ground flaxseed, chocolate chips, and a little bit of salt.

Mix the wet ingredients.
Mix the nut butter, honey maple syrup, and vanilla extract with the dry ingredients. Stir until everything is mixed well.

Stir together really well.
Use a cooking tool or your hands to carefully mix all the ingredients. The mixture needs to be sticky and stay in one piece.

Cool down the mixture:
Put the mix in the fridge for 30 minutes to make it easier to work with.

Shape Bites:
After you have let the mixture cool, use your hands to make small balls out of it. You can pick any size you want but try to make it about 1 inch across.

Store:

Put the protein bites on a tray or plate lined with parchment paper and put them in the fridge for at least 30 more minutes to harden.
Have fun:

Once the protein bites are hard, put them in a sealed container and keep them in the fridge. Grab a few when you need a fast energy boost.

Tips :
Chop up some nuts like almonds, walnuts, or pistachios, or sprinkle some seeds like chia or sunflower seeds for more crunch and nutrition.

Add cut-up dried fruits like raisins, cranberries, or apricots for a sweet taste.

Sprinkle some unsweetened coconut flakes on the protein bites for more taste.

Spices: Put a little bit of cinnamon or nutmeg for a cozy and fragrant taste.

These protein bites give you energy and are sweet. They have protein, healthy fats, and complex carbs to keep you going. They are a handy and easy-to-carry snack to give you energy all day long.

CHAPTER SEVEN

HYDRATION STATION

It's really important to drink enough water to stay healthy and feel good. Here are some ideas for drinks that you can make at home to stay hydrated.

Recipes for flavored water
Flavored water is a nice and refreshing way to keep your body hydrated without sugary or fake tastes. Here are some ideas for flavored water to make your drinks taste better and help you stay hydrated.

Water that has been flavored with cucumber, mint, and lime.
Half of a cucumber is cut into thin round pieces.
A few fresh mint leaves
1 lime, cut into thin slices.
15 liters of water means one and a half liters of water.

Steps:
Put cucumber slices, mint leaves, and lime slices in a pitcher.
Put water in the pitcher and cool it in the fridge for at least 2 hours before you use it.

Berry Citrus Flavored Water:
1 cup of different types of berries (strawberries, blueberries, raspberries)
One orange, cut into pieces.
1 lemon, cut into thin pieces.
15 liters of water means one big bottle of water.

Instructions:
Put some different berries, orange slices, and lemon slices in a big container.
Put water in the fridge for a couple of hours so the flavors mix.

Refreshing water is made by soaking watermelon and basil in it.
2 cups of chopped watermelon.
A few fresh basil leaves
1. 5 liters of water means a big bottle of water.

How to do something:
Mix pieces of watermelon and basil leaves in a large container.
Put water in the pitcher and put it in the fridge to get cold. Pour over ice.

A drink made with pineapple and coconut flavors mixed with water.
1 cup of chopped pineapple
Half a cup of pieces of coconut or liquid from inside a coconut.
15 liters of water is equal to about 6 cups of water.

Direction
Combine pieces of pineapple and pieces of coconut, or coconut water, in a pitcher.
Put water in and place it in the refrigerator for a delicious tropical treat.

Ginger, lemon, and honey mixed in water.
Cut one lemon into thin slices.
A small slice of fresh ginger, about one inch long.
1 spoon of honey
1. 5 liters of water means one and a half liters of water.

How to do something:
Put lemon slices and ginger slices in a pitcher.
Mix honey with the water. Mix thoroughly and leave it in the fridge to soak.

Raspberry Rosemary Water:
1 measure of fresh raspberries
Two small branches of fresh rosemary.
15 liters of water means one and a half liters of water.

How to do something:
Mix raspberries and rosemary in a jug.
Put water in the pitcher and then put it in the fridge to make a tasty flavored drink.
Suggestions for Flavored Water:
Let the water sit for at least 2 hours or overnight to make the flavors stronger.
Please feel free to change the amount of ingredients to fit your taste.
You can add more water to the pitcher a few times before putting in new fruits and herbs.

Flavored water not only tastes good but also gives you extra vitamins and antioxidants from the fruits and herbs. Try different things and combine them to find the mix of flavors you like best.

Relaxing Herbal Teas
Herbal teas can help you relax and feel calm. Here are some herbal teas that are famous for helping you feel relaxed.

Chamomile tea:
Chamomile is well-known for making you feel calm and relaxed. It can make you feel less worried and help you sleep better. Relax with a cup of tea or coffee at night.

Peppermint tea:
Peppermint tea tastes good and can help you feel relaxed. This can reduce stress and make your muscles feel better. It also helps digestion.

lavender Tea:
Lavender can help you feel calm and relaxed. Make a cup of lavender tea to feel less stressed and more relaxed. You might want to add a little honey for sweetness.

Valerian root Tea.
Valerian root is often used as a natural way to help with sleeping problems and feeling worried or stressed. It tastes strong and earthy and is best to eat before going to bed.

Lemon Balm Tea:
Lemon balm is a type of mint plant that can help you relax. It tastes like lemons and can help you feel less stressed and anxious.

Passionflower Tea:
Passionflower is used to help people relax and sleep better. It tastes mild and is often mixed with other herbs that help you relax.

Rosehip tea:
Rosehip tea has lots of vitamin C and antioxidants. It tastes a little sour and can help you feel calm and boost your immune system when you drink it.

Hibiscus tea.
Hibiscus tea is bright red and tastes tangy. It is well-liked for its calming and refreshing effects and is often enjoyed as a cold tea.

Green tea without caffeine.
Green tea without caffeine has L-theanine, an amino acid that helps you relax without making you tired. It also gives a gentle caffeine option.

Fruit-Infused Sparkling Water
Fruit-infused sparkling water is a tasty and healthy option instead of sugary sodas and juices that can help keep you hydrated. Here's an easy way to make your own flavored sparkling water with fruit at home:

Ingredients:

Bubbly water (plain or with added flavors, as you like).
Different types of fruits (such as berries, citrus slices, and melon cubes)

Fresh herbs like mint and basil.
Ice cubes
Directions:
Get the fruits and herbs ready:
Clean and cut the fruits. Cut citrus fruits into thin slices. You can either keep berries whole or cut larger ones in half. Choose, new herbs like mint or basil.

Choose Your Sparkling Water:
Choose the sparkling water you like the most. You can choose plain sparkling water or flavored ones, based on what you like.

Mix the ingredients.
In a big pitcher or separate glasses, mix the cut fruits and herbs. Put ice cubes to make it extra cold.

Sparkling Water for pouring:
Put the fizzy water on top of the fruits and herbs. If you are using a pitcher, stir slowly to mix the things inside.

Let it soak in.
Let the fruit and herb mixture sit for 5-10 minutes to soak up the flavors. The flavor becomes more intense the longer you wait.

Serve and have fun:
Pour the fizzy water with fruit flavor into glasses, making sure each serving has some fruit and herbs in it. You can remove any chunks from the water if you want it to be smoother.

Different Flavors to Mix:
Citrus Burst: A citrusy flavor explosion.
Pieces of oranges, lemons, and limes with a fresh mint leaf.

Delightful berries:

Different types of berries like strawberries, blueberries, and raspberries with a little bit of basil.

Beautiful tropical island:
Pieces of pineapple, slices of mango, and a little bit of fresh cilantro leaves.

Refresh yourself with this tasty and healthy drink made from cucumber and melon. Ready to enjoy?
Slices of cucumber mixed with chunks of watermelon and a little bit of mint.

Apple Spice Refresher: A drink made with apple and spices, that is refreshing and full of flavor.
Thinly sliced apples and a few cinnamon sticks to make a warm fall drink.

Grapefruit Rosemary Twist: A drink made with grapefruit and rosemary.
Slices of grapefruit with rosemary for a fancy taste.

Advice: Make the text easier.
Change the amount of fruit to match how much you like it.
Combine different fruits and herbs to make special flavor combinations.
Make sparkling water at home by using a soda maker.
This tasty sparkling water with fruit flavor is better for you than sugary drinks. It's a drink that you can change to fit your likes, and you can have it at any time of the year.

CHAPTER EIGHT

DESSERTS WITH A TWIST

Making desserts differently lets you try new flavors, textures, and ways to show them. Here are some special dessert ideas to make your sweet treats more creative.

Berry Sorbet with Mint:
Mixed berry dessert with fresh mint flavor.
Berry sorbet with mint is a cool and sweet dessert made from berries and mint. Here's an easy way to make delicious berry sorbet with mint:

Ingredients:
3 cups of mixed berries like strawberries, blueberries, and raspberries.
1/2 cup of white sugar (depending on how sweet you want it)
1/4 cup of mint leaves from the plant
2 tablespoons of freshly squeezed lemon juice
1 measure of water.

Instructions:
Get the berries ready:

Clean the berries well and take off any stems.

Make sweet syrup:
Mix the sugar and water in a pot. Warm the mixture on medium heat and stir until the sugar disappears. Allow it to cool down until it's no longer warm.
Mix the ingredients.
Put the mixed berries, mint leaves, and fresh lemon juice into a blender and mix them. Add the cold sugar water to the mix.

Mix until no lumps are left:
Mix the ingredients until they are smooth and fully mixed.

Strain (Optional):
If you want your sorbet to be smoother, you can pour the mixture through a strainer to take out the seeds and pulp. Use a small-holed strainer or a piece of cloth to strain.

Cool down the mixture.
Put the berry mix in the fridge for at least 2 hours or until it's very cold.

Put into the ice cream maker and allow to freeze.
Put the cold mixture into an ice cream maker and follow the instructions from the maker.

Use immediately or put in the freezer.
As soon as the sorbet becomes like soft ice cream, you can serve it right away. To make the sorbet firmer, put it in a closed container and freeze it for a few hours.

Top with mint leaves:
Before you serve it, put some fresh mint leaves on top of the berry sorbet to make it smell and look even better.
Have fun:

Put the berry sorbet into bowls or cones and enjoy the yummy mix of sweet berries and mint.

Tips: Here are some helpful suggestions:
Change how sweet it is by putting in more or less sugar depending on how you like it.

You can choose which fruits you want in the berry mix.
If you don't have an ice cream maker, you can pour the mixture into a flat dish, put it in the freezer, and use a fork to scrape it into a texture like granita.
This minty berry frozen dessert is a tasty way to savor the flavors of summer. It's refreshing, fruity, and great for when it's hot outside.

Strawberries covered in dark chocolate.

Strawberries covered in dark chocolate are a fancy dessert that combines the sweetness of strawberries with rich dark chocolate. Here's an easy recipe to make this tasty treat:

Ingredients:
Clean and dry fresh strawberries.
Cut about 8 ounces of dark chocolate.
White chocolate (you can add it if you like for decoration)
Toppings like nuts, coconut, or sprinkles are optional.

Instructions:
Get the strawberries ready:
Make sure to wash and dry the strawberries completely. Leaving the stems on can make it easier to hold them.

Dark chocolate needs to be heated until it becomes liquid.
Melt the dark chocolate in a bowl, either using a double boiler or a microwave. Keep stirring every 20 seconds until it becomes smooth.

Put the strawberries in the liquid.
Grab each strawberry by the green part and dip it in the melted dark chocolate, making sure it's all covered. Let extra chocolate drip off.

Put the parchment paper down.
Put the strawberries that have been dipped in chocolate on a tray lined

with parchment paper. This stops them from getting stuck and makes it easier to clean up.

Choose what you want to put on top.
While the chocolate is still soft, put toppings like nuts, coconut, or sprinkles on the strawberries. This will give them an even more enjoyable taste.

Allow them to sit down.
Let the chocolate-covered strawberries sit at room temperature. You can make it faster by putting the tray in the fridge for 15-20 minutes.

An extra topping of white chocolate sauce is available if wanted.
If you want to, you can melt the white chocolate using the same method as the dark chocolate. Pour the melted white chocolate over the hardened dark chocolate using a spoon or a piping bag.

The last part of the story:
Let the white chocolate sauce harden before you serve it.

Use and have fun:
Put the strawberries dipped in chocolate on a plate and have this yummy and fancy dessert.

Tips:
Use good dark chocolate for the best taste.
Try different things on top of your chocolate-covered strawberries to make them look different and more colorful.

If you're serving them for a special event, think about putting them in a pretty box or on a fancy plate.
Dipping strawberries in dark chocolate makes them a yummy treat that looks nice. They're great for parties, date nights, or just when you want something sweet.

Coconut Chia Pudding

Coconut chia pudding is a yummy and healthy treat you can eat for dessert or breakfast. It has the smooth taste of coconut milk and the good stuff found in chia seeds. Here's an easy way to make coconut chia pudding:

Ingredients:
1/4 cup of chia seeds
1 cup of coconut milk from a can (use full-fat for a creamier texture)
1 or 2 tablespoons of maple syrup or any desired sweetener.
1/2 teaspoon of vanilla flavoring
You can choose to add shredded coconut, fresh berries, sliced bananas, or nuts on top.

Instructions:
Mix things:
Mix chia seeds, coconut milk, maple syrup, and vanilla in a bowl or jar.

Mix thoroughly
Mix the chia seeds well so they are spread out evenly and don't stick together.

Allow it to rest or settle:
Put a lid on the bowl or jar and put it in the fridge for at least 4 hours or, even better, overnight. This lets the chia seeds soak up the liquid and turn into a thick pudding.

Mix again (if you want to).
Once the mixture has set for a while, stir it again to break up any clumps that might be there.

Taste the sweetness:
Try the pudding and if it's not sweet enough, add more maple syrup to make it sweeter.

Serve:
Put the coconut chia pudding into bowls or jars.

Add Toppings:
Put the toppings you like on the pudding, like coconut, berries, bananas, or nuts.

Have fun:
Have and eat your delicious and healthy coconut chia pudding.

Tips:
Try using different amounts of chia seeds and coconut milk to get the thickness you want.
If you like coconut milk to be smooth, mix it with other ingredients first before you add the chia seeds.

Change how sweet it is by putting in more or less maple syrup until it tastes good to you.
Coconut chia pudding tastes great and is good for you because it has lots of fiber, healthy fats, and protein from plants. It's a flexible recipe that you can change with different toppings to fit your tastes.

CHAPTER NINE

RECIPES FOR SPECIAL OCCASIONS.

On special days, it's nice to make recipes that taste great and look fancy. Here are some special recipes for special occasions that you might like:

Simple Quinoa Salad for a Party
A colorful and healthy quinoa salad is great for parties and special events. This salad has lots of different colorful vegetables, herbs, and a tasty dressing. It not only tastes great but also looks pretty. Here is a recipe for a special quinoa salad:

Ingredients:
For the salad:
1 cup of quinoa, washed and cooked as directed on the package.
1 cup of small tomatoes that have been cut in half.
1 cucumber, cut into small pieces
Cut 1 red bell pepper into smaller pieces.
One yellow bell pepper, cut into small pieces.
1 cup of carrots that have been cut into thin strips
1/2 cup of red onion that has been cut into very small pieces.

1/2 cup of fresh cilantro that has been cut into small pieces.
1/2 cup of chopped fresh mint leaves.
1 cup of crumbled feta cheese, if you like it

For the sauce:
1/4 cup of very good olive oil
3 spoons of balsamic vinegar
1 spoon of Dijon mustard
1 piece of garlic, chopped into very tiny pieces
Sprinkle some salt and black pepper according to your liking.

Directions:
Make Quinoa:
Wash quinoa with cold water and cook it as directed on the package. Let it cool completely.

Prepare the dressing.
Mix olive oil, balsamic vinegar, Dijon mustard, minced garlic, salt, and black pepper in a small bowl. Put to the side.

Make the salad:
In a big bowl, mix cooked and cooled quinoa with cherry tomatoes, cucumber, red and yellow bell peppers, shredded carrots, red onion, cilantro, and mint.

Add Dressing:
Drizzle the dressing on the salad and mix it gently to make sure the quinoa and veggies are covered.

Sprinkle some Feta cheese on top if you want.
If you have feta cheese, break it into small pieces and sprinkle it on top of the salad. Then, mix it all gently.

Cool and then dish it out.
Put the quinoa salad in the fridge for at least 30 minutes so that the flavors can mix. This salad can be eaten cold.

Optional extra decoration:
Before you finish making the food, you can add some extra fresh herbs or a little bit of feta on top.

Serve and Enjoy: To do something for others and take pleasure in it.
Offer the Celebration Quinoa Salad as a colorful and healthy side dish for your special party.

Hints:
Change the vegetables depending on what is in season or what you like.
You can add grilled chicken, shrimp, or tofu to get more protein.
Change the ingredients in the dressing until it tastes just right - not too sweet and not too sour.

This Celebration Quinoa Salad is not only beautiful but also healthy and filling for your special events.

Grilled chicken on sticks with special sauce.

Grilled chicken on sticks with a mustard sauce is a tasty and juicy dish that's great for parties. The marinade makes the grilled chicken taste tangy and delicious. Here's how to make Grilled Chicken Skewers with Dijon Marinade:

Ingredients:
To make the marinade:
- 1/4 cup of Dijon mustard
2 spoons of honey
2 tablespoons of olive oil
2 pieces of garlic, finely chopped
1 small spoon of dried thyme
1 teaspoon of dried rosemary leaves.
Add as little or as much salt and black pepper as you want.

To make the chicken skewers:
1. 5 pounds of chicken breasts without bones or skin, cut into small pieces.
If you're using wooden sticks, put them in water for 30 minutes before grilling.

Optional topping:
Chopped fresh parsley.
Slices of lemon

Instructions:
Make the marinade:
Mix Dijon mustard, honey, olive oil, minced garlic, thyme, rosemary, salt, and pepper in a bowl.

Soak chicken in a seasoning sauce.
Put the pieces of chicken in a flat dish or a plastic bag that can be sealed. Pour the Dijon sauce over the chicken so that all pieces are covered well. Chill in the fridge for 30 minutes so the flavors mix.

Preheat the grill: Start heating the grill.
Start up your grill and set it to a medium-high temperature.

Chicken on a stick:
Put the chicken cubes that have been soaked in marinade onto the skewers, making sure to leave a small gap between each piece.

Cook the skewers on the grill.
Cook the chicken on a grill for 8-10 minutes, turning it every so often, until it's fully cooked and has a yummy crispy edge.

See if it's cooked enough:
Make sure the inside of the chicken is heated to 165°F (74°C).

Relax and decorate.
Let the grilled chicken skewers sit for a few minutes before you eat them. Sprinkle with chopped parsley and put lemon wedges next to it when you serve.

Serve and have fun:
Put the grilled chicken on a plate and serve it while it's still hot. They taste good with rice, quinoa, or a salad.

Advice:
You can put a little bit of lemon juice in the marinade to give it a tangy citrus flavor.
Try using different herbs and spices like paprika or cayenne pepper in the marinade to create new flavors.
Serve the skewers with a side of tzatziki sauce or a yogurt dip to make them more creamy.

These Grilled Chicken Skewers with Dijon Marinade will be a big hit at any party. They have a delicious mix of sweet, savory, and herby flavors.

Festive Fruit Salad
A fruit salad is a nice and refreshing dish for parties and celebrations. Here's how to make a yummy fruit salad with different fruits and a citrus dressing.

Ingredients:
To make the fruit salad:
2 cups of strawberries, with the stems removed and cut in half.
1 measuring cup of blueberries
1 cup of green grapes, cut in half.
1 cup of pineapple pieces
1 kiwi, without the skin, cut into pieces
1 cup of peeled and broken-down mandarin oranges
1 cup of pomegranate seeds

Garnish with fresh mint leaves.
To make the citrus dressing:
A quarter cup of orange juice
2 spoons of honey

1 spoonful of lime juice
Juice from 1 lime
One small spoon of poppy seeds (if you want)

Instructions:

Make the Citrus Dressing:
Mix orange juice, honey, lime juice, lime zest, and poppy seeds (if using) in a small bowl. Put aside

Make the Fruit Salad:
Put the strawberries, blueberries, green grapes, pineapple chunks, kiwi slices, mandarin orange segments, and pomegranate arils in a big bowl.

Pour the dressing over the food
Put the lemony sauce on top of the fruit mix. Gently mix the fruits with the dressing.

Chill:
Put the fruit salad in the fridge for at least 30 minutes so the flavors can mix and the salad can get cold.

Garnish
Before you serve the fruit salad, add some fresh mint leaves on top for a burst of fresh flavor.

Serve:
Put the fruit salad in bowls or on a big plate.

Have fun:
Offer the fruit salad as a colorful and healthy treat for your special event.

Tips:
Choose the fruits you like from the available options and consider what fruits are in season.
Sprinkle a few toasted coconut flakes or chopped nuts for more crunch.
If you're making the fruit salad ahead of time, wait until right before you serve it to add the dressing. This will help the fruit stay fresh and crunchy.

This fruit salad looks great and has lots of tasty flavors. It will make your taste buds happy. It's a refreshing choice that goes well with different dishes for special events.

CHAPTER TEN

KITCHEN TIPS AND TECHNIQUES

Kitchen tips are helpful advice and skills for cooking and preparing food. These tips and techniques are designed to help you cook better and have more fun while doing it.

Simple changes in cooking for people with Alzheimer's disease
Taking care of people with Alzheimer's disease means changing how we cook and what we cook to make sure it's safe, easy, and enjoyable for them. Here are some simple changes to recipes for people with Alzheimer's disease to make cooking easier.

1. Simple Recipes:
Choose easy recipes with only a few ingredients and easy steps. Pay attention to the dishes that you already know and love.

2. Preparation Assistance:
Help with things like cutting, measuring, and mixing. Cut the veggies beforehand and have all ingredients ready to use.

3. Visual Aids:

Use pictures or word labels to help understand the steps or what is in the ingredients. This makes it simple to recognize and understand.

4. Instructions in one step:
Divide tasks into small steps and only give one direction at a time. This helps people with Alzheimer's understand better.

5. Kitchen Safety:
Make sure the kitchen is safe. Get rid of stuff you don't need, keep your walkways open, and don't leave things lying around.

6. Easier to hold utensils:
Provide utensils with handles that are comfortable to hold and easy to use. This can help you be more independent when you are making meals.

7. Adapted Cooking Tools:
Use kitchen tools that are easy to use and adjust to your needs, like can openers, timers, and measuring cups with big letters.

8. Slow Cooker or Instant Pot Meals:
Make cooking easier by using slow cookers or Instant Pots. These machines need very little help and can make tasty food.

9. Finger foods:
Try making meals that you can eat with your hands so you don't have to use utensils.

Safety rules for the kitchen
It is very important to keep the kitchen safe to avoid accidents and injuries. Here are some important things to do to stay safe in the kitchen:

1. Keep things clean:
Clean your countertops, cutting boards, and utensils often to avoid spreading germs.

2. Handling food correctly:
Wash your hands well before touching food. Keep uncooked meat away from foods that you can eat without cooking, and use separate cutting

boards for each.

3. The temperatures that are safe for cooking.
Make sure to cook meats to their right temperatures inside to get rid of any bad germs. Use a food thermometer to check that food is cooked properly.

4. Fire Safety:
It's important to be safe and prepared in case of a fire.
Don't put things that can catch on fire near the stove. Store a fire-fighting device in the kitchen and make sure you know how to operate it.

5 Avoid getting burned:
Use thick gloves when touching hot pots and pans. Be careful around steam and hot surfaces. Turn the handles of the pots away from the front of the stove.

6. Knife Safety:
Keep your knives sharp so you can control them better. Make sure you cut things the right way and stay focused when chopping.

7 . Electrical Safety:
Check the cords for any signs of wear and tear. Only plug a few things into one outlet and always unplug things when you are not using them.

8. Slip and Fall Prevention:
Make sure the floors are not wet, and if anything spills, clean it up right away. Put non-slip rugs by the sink and stove.

9. Child Safety:
Keep dangerous things like knives, chemicals, and other harmful objects away from kids where they can't reach them. Put locks on cabinets to keep them safe.

Planning and Preparing Meals Effectively
Making good plans and getting ready to cook meals smartly can help you save time and money, and make sure you eat healthy and tasty food. Here

are some helpful ideas for planning and making meals.

Meal Planning:
Plan out the meals you will eat for the entire week.
Make a plan for what you want to eat each day for the next week. Use different types of proteins, vegetables, grains, and fruits.

Think about what you eat.

Consider any special diets, likes, or health goals when making meal plans.

"Make sure to check in the pantry and fridge. "
Before you go to the store, make sure to see what food you already have at home. This helps to stop buying too much and throwing away less food.

Batch cooking
Instead of cooking one meal at a time, you cook many meals and then store them for later.

Try cooking a lot of one thing, like grains or meat, and then use it in different meals all week.

Simple Recipes that can be changed to fit different ingredients or preferences.
Select recipes that can be changed with different ingredients. This can be useful if you have extra food or need to use certain ingredients.

Ingredients that save time.
Use pre-cut vegetables, canned beans, and frozen fruits to save time when cooking.

List of items needed for grocery shopping:
Create a list of everything you need to buy for your meals. Include all the details of what you'll need. Follow the list so you don't buy things on a whim.

Prepare the ingredients ahead of time.

Prepare the ingredients ahead of time by washing, cutting, and measuring them into portions. Please put them in the fridge so it's easy to get to them during the week.

Making food:
Organizing the kitchen:
Make sure your kitchen is neat. Organize your tools and ingredients so that you can work easily.

Begin with a tidy kitchen:
Start cooking in a kitchen that is clean and tidy. It makes things more fun and gives a good feeling.

Stick to a plan for cooking.
Create a plan for cooking that says when each part of the meal will be made. This helps you to manage your time effectively.

Doing multiple things at once.
Find tasks that can be done at the same time to make cooking faster. For instance, when something is cooking, you can make a salad.

Easy to make meals where all the ingredients are cooked in just one pan. Choose to make meals using only one pan or one pot to make cleaning up easier and cooking simpler.

Cooking in large quantities at once.
If you can, make more food and put some in the freezer for later. This is very helpful for days when you are very busy.

Clean as you go
Clean counters and wash dishes while you cook to keep your kitchen clean. It helps clean up after a meal easier.

Eating smaller amounts of food:
Be mindful of how much food you serve to avoid cooking too much and throwing away leftovers. Use tools to measure if necessary.

Buy tools that help you do things faster.
Use items like slow cookers, Instant Pots, or food processors in the kitchen to make some tasks faster.

Enjoy the journey:
Think of making meals as a fun and creative thing to do. Listen to music or spend time with your family for a good time.

By using these tips to plan and prepare meals, you can make cooking easier, save time, and make sure your meals are tasty and healthy.

CHAPTER ELEVEN

CAREGIVER'S CORNER

The "Caregiver's Corner" is a special place for caregivers to get help and information about taking care of others. It can be physical or online. This place can help caregivers do their job better by providing different tools and information. Here are some things that could be in a caregiver's corner:

The Role of Nutrition in Alzheimer's Care
Eating healthy food is very important for people with Alzheimer's. It helps to keep their body and brain healthy. Eating the right food can make you feel better, help your brain work better, and might make a disease go slower. Here are important parts of how food helps people with Alzheimer's:

Brain-Healthy Nutrients:
Eating foods that are good for your brain is important. These are healthy things in food like fish and fruits and vegetables that help your body.

Brain-Healthy Nutrients:
Try to eat a mix of fruits, veggies, whole grains, lean meats, and good fats

to stay healthy. This gives important nutrients for good health.

Keeping your body hydrated :
Drinking enough water is very important. Not drinking enough water can make confusion worse and cause other health problems. Encourage drinking water often and offer foods like fruits and soups that keep the body hydrated.

Weight Management:
Controlling and keeping track of your body weight.
It's important to keep a healthy weight. Collaborate with doctors to keep track of your weight and make changes to your diet as needed.

Changed Texture and Appearance:
As Alzheimer's gets worse, people may have trouble chewing or swallowing. Change the way food looks or make it look really good so that it makes people want to eat it and enjoy it.

Eating small meals regularly.
Instead of eating big meals, try eating smaller meals more often. This can make it easier for people with Alzheimer's to handle and process.

Avoid eating too much processed food.
Eat less processed foods that have a lot of unhealthy fats and sugars. Choose food that is good for you and has lots of vitamins and minerals.

Taking extra vitamins or minerals.
If needed, think about taking extra vitamins or minerals. Talk to doctors or other health experts to find out if taking certain vitamins or supplements like vitamin D or omega-3 can be helpful for you.

Catering to Different Diets:
Please tell us if you have any specific dietary needs or restrictions, like if you have diabetes or heart problems. Collaborate with doctors and nutrition experts.

Tips for Encouraging Healthy Eating Habits
Creating a positive and supportive environment is important for encouraging healthy eating habits and promoting good nutrition. Here are some tips for fostering healthy eating habits, whether it's for yourself, your family, or individuals under your care:

Lead by Example:
Show good eating habits by including different healthy foods in your meals. Kids and people who are taken care of usually copy what adults do.

Provide access to healthy foods.
Make sure to have different types of fresh fruits, vegetables, whole grains, and lean proteins in your kitchen where you can see them easily. This makes it simple to make healthy choices.

Include everyone in deciding what to eat for meals.
Involve your family or the people you take care of in planning meals together. Find out what people like and then include their favorite healthy foods.

Let's cook together.
Cooking with others can be a fun way to learn and have a good time. Include everyone in tasks that are suitable for their age, so they feel proud and connected to the food.

Be imaginative with how you present things.
Present food in an attractive way. Put different colored fruits and vegetables on a plate or try decorating them in fun ways to make healthy food look more attractive.

Introduce new foods slowly.
Take your time and be patient when trying new foods. It can take time for people, especially kids, to like new foods.

Avoid drinking sugary drinks, like soda and sweetened juice, too often.
Encourage drinking water instead of other drinks. Don't drink too many sugary drinks like sodas and fruit juices. Try adding fruits or herbs to your

water to make it taste better.

Have your food same time daily.
Set the same times each day for meals to make a schedule. This helps control how hungry you feel and encourages paying attention to what you eat.

Eat less processed foods.
Eat less processed and fast foods. Choose natural, unprocessed foods that have lots of good nutrients.

Balancing Nutrition and Enjoyment
It's important to eat food that is good for you and that you like, to stay healthy and keep going. Here
are some ideas to help you find the right mix:

Eat more healthy foods:
Fruits, vegetables, whole grains, and lean proteins.
Choose healthy foods that have a lot of nutrients for your meals. These are foods like fruits, vegetables, whole grains, lean meats, and good fats.

Enjoy different types of foods:
Eat many different types of food to make sure you get all the nutrients you need. Try using different types of fruits, vegetables, and whole grains to make meals more exciting.

Practice using moderation:
Eat a little bit of all types of food. It's okay to sometimes eat unhealthy food as long as you also eat healthy food most of the time.

Listen to Your Body:

Remember to listen to your body when it's telling you if you're hungry or full. Consume food only when you feel hunger and cease eating when you feel satiated." Eat the right amount.

Enjoy the Tastes:
Take your time and enjoy your food when you eat. Eating mindfully means enjoying the taste, feel, and smell of your food.

Cook and Explore New Recipes:
Make cooking fun and pleasant. Try new recipes, mix different flavors, and cook with your friends or family.

Balance Macro-nutrients:
Keep a healthy balance of protein, carbohydrates, and fats in your diet.
Ensure to mix of crabs, proteins, and fats in your meals.
Every type of nutrient is important for keeping the body healthy.

Use treats carefully:
If you have a favorite snack or food that makes you feel good, make sure to eat it thoughtfully. Enjoy the experience without feeling bad.

Remember to drink plenty of water.
Drinking more water is very important for staying healthy. Remember to drink water all day long, and you can also add fruits or herbs to make it tastier.

CHAPTER TWELVE

CONCLUSION

In summary, there is no specific diet for Alzheimer's. But eating a variety of healthy foods seems to be good for the brain and overall health. Eating fruits, veggies, whole grains, lean meats, and healthy fats is good for your heart and might help your brain too.

It's really important to think about what you eat as part of taking care of someone with Alzheimer's. It's also important to make sure they are active, spend time with others, and get good medical care. Also, personalized meal plans should take into account specific health problems, likes and dislikes, and how food might affect medications.

As scientists learn more about how food affects Alzheimer's, it's important to stay updated and talk to health care experts, like dietitians, for the best advice on eating for brain health. This can help people with Alzheimer's and also those who want to keep their brains healthy. In general, taking care of a person with Alzheimer's, including their diet, can help them and their caregivers have a better life.

www.ingramcontent.com/pod-product-compliance
Lightning Source LLC
Chambersburg PA
CBHW070411230526
45471CB00006B/2761